T0208320

Healing Journeys

My Path to Freedom

Mary Abdool-Warner

BALBOA.
PRESS
A DIVISION OF HAY HOUSE

Balboa Press books may be ordered through booksellers or by contacting:

Balboa Press
A Division of Hay House
1663 Liberty Drive
Bloomington, IN 47403
www.balboapress.com
1 (877) 407-4847

Print information available on the last page.

ISBN: 978-1-9822-3093-7 (sc)
ISBN: 978-1-9822-3094-4 (e)

Balboa Press rev. date: 12/05/2019

Contents

Introduction

HEALING: The Joys and Pain of My Healing

I got healed of Carpal Tunnel Syndrome without surgery. It was a long process but I avoided surgery against my doctor's wishes. I took control of my life. I took matters into my own hands and I'm glad I did. That was back in 2012. I knew nothing about pain except for labour pain twice in my life. As for healing, I had never experienced it, neither did I know anyone who had experienced any form of healing.

I think we're often learning more than we realize as we live our lives. Looking back, it surprises me to think how much more I know today than I did even five or ten years ago. On a day to day basis, I'd never know how much I was internalizing. I have learned a lot about healing since then and I'm still learning. There is so much information out there about every disease you can think of. I developed a passion for learning about healing. Passion is the fuel that drives us forward in life: the passion to experience, to create value, to invent, to build something that has a life of its own. To connect with other people, but best of all, to do something remarkable with our lives- whatever it is that's important to us. My healing took place gradually in 2016, after years of physio-therapy with no relief from the pain. Then after specific prayers from cherished friends and believers like myself, the pain finally vanished and my skin returned to its normal colour. Non-traditional doctors and laypeople alike willingly share their knowledge. Much of it from their own experiences and that of others. That's what prompted me to write this book. I want other people to know that they too can heal and go on to lead a healthy, normal life without being operated on, only to later discover that the problem returns. Surgery is not necessarily a cure-all for all illnesses.

Chapter 1
What Is Carpal Tunnel?

It is a narrow passageway on the palm side of your wrist made up of bones and ligaments. The median nerve, which controls sensation and movement in the thumb and first three fingers, runs through this passageway along with tendons to the fingers and thumb. When it is pinched or compressed, the result is numbness, tingling, weakness, or pain in the hand, called Carpal Tunnel Syndrome. Carpal Tunnel develops slowly. At first, you're most likely to notice it at night or when you first wake up in the morning. The feeling is similar to "pins and needles" sensation you get when your hand falls asleep. Coping with carpal tunnel symptoms can be frustrating. You use your hands in so many ways that it inhibits many of life's tasks and pleasures to having numbness and weakness. During the day, you will notice pain or tingling when holding things like a phone or a book, and in my case when driving. Shaking or moving your fingers usually help. As Carpal Tunnel Syndrome progresses, you may begin to notice weakness in the thumb and first two fingers, and it may be difficult to make a fist or grasp objects. You may find yourself dropping things or you may have trouble doing things like holding a utensil or buttoning your shirt. This caused me to become so helpless, that my daughter had to come over every other day after work to wash my dishes. That was embarrassing since it went on for a long time, but I thank God for the help I received from her. Some people feel like their fingers are swollen, even though no swelling is present, or they may have trouble distinguishing between hot and cold.

ROOT CAUSES OF CARPAL TUNNEL AND OTHER DISEASES

There usually isn't one definite cause for Carpal Tunnel Syndrome. Because the carpal tunnel is narrow and rigid, anytime there is swelling or inflammation in the area, the median nerve can be compressed and cause pain. Symptoms may be present in one or both hands. Usually symptoms develop in the dominant hand first. Women are three times more likely than men to get Carpal Tunnel Syndrome. Certain conditions can also increase your risk. These include: Diabetes, gout, hypothyroidism, rheumatoid arthritis, pregnancy, sprain or fractured wrist.

I mentioned that my skin returned to its normal colour. I don't know what caused the discolouration in my left hand, but it gradually changed from brown to white. That was so embarrassing for me that I hid my hand under long sleeved tops. I thought I had contracted leprosy. From what I've heard about leprosy, it is an infectious disease caused by a bacterium. If left untreated, leprosy can have devastating effects. The disease can create health problems and physical impairment. Because it is still feared, many affected face long-lasting mental health issues and social stigma. Although leprosy is a disease that has been around for millennia, we still need to learn more. Even though we have a drug therapy that treats the disease, hundreds of thousands of people with leprosy continue to be diagnosed each year. There are millions alive today that live with disability, poverty and isolation because of leprosy. This disease causes unbearable itching, skin discolouration, lesions and blindness if untreated. It is painful and disfigures various parts of the body. The disease is caused by exposure to Mycobacterium Leptae, a bacteria that grows slowly in the body once a person has been exposed. The condition may also be called Hansen's disease, named after the scientist credited for discovering M. Lepme in 1873. Since the bacteria grows slowly, it can take three to five years for symptoms to develop after a person has been exposed. In some cases it can even take up to twenty years for symptoms to develop.

Some early signs of Leprosy.

- Numbness in the affected areas. Usually in the hands and feet, spreading to the arms and legs
- Loss of temperature sensation: The inability to sense changes in temperature
- Pins and needles sensation. It's characterized by tingling or prickling of the skin
- Pain. As the nerves are affected by the bacteria, it causes pain
- Deep pressure sensation. Causes clumsiness or accident prone
- Nerve injury. This process begins to cause deformities and a burning sensation in the skin
- Weight loss
- Blisters. Often begins with a red patch of skin similar to a rash but continues to worsen
- Ulcers. As blisters worsen, they begin to develop into open sores
- Skin Lesions. These can be flat, raised, lightly coloured or darker

As you can see, those suffering from carpal tunnel may experience similar symptoms as in the early stages of leprosy.

PAIN

There are numerous underlying causes of pain. It may be physical pain from an injury or chronic illness, mental and emotional pain such as anxiety or depression, or the exhausting and often constant stress from binge eating and trying to control your weight. Acute pain is a short term form of pain. When you have an accident, acute injury, illness or surgery, you may experience sudden and often more severe pain. In most cases, acute pain goes away within a few hours, days, or weeks without treatment depending on the cause of your pain. In some cases, acute pain may turn chronic.

Chronic pain is a more persistent pain that can lasts for months or even years. In some cases, chronic pain occurs after an illness or injury when the pain lingers even after the health issue is resolved. In other cases, chronic pain is due to a chronic health condition, inflammation or overuse injury. The source of chronic pain can be a very complex and even mysterious issue to talk about. It is resistant to most medical treatments and can cause severe problems. I guess my pain was somewhere in the middle. Not acute but not too chronic.

MEDICATIONS

When symptoms and pain are more severe, your doctor may recommend corticosteroids by injection or mouth. Steroids can temporarily reduce inflammation around the median nerve and ease symptoms. My doctor recommended me to a specialist who would give me a cortisone shot in my left wrist. I was in so much pain that I agreed to have the procedure done. I have a high pain tolerance so I did not think about the pain I would get from the needle. On the morning of the procedure, I almost fainted when I saw the size of the needle. I looked away when the needle was inserted into the skin. My pain tolerance evaporated in thin air. All I heard the specialist say was, "Keep your hand still". I wondered how much longer I could stand that pain and keep my hand still, but she kept on pushing the needle deeper. Just when I thought I would faint, she said," It is in". She pumped the medicine in and pulled out the needle. The act of the needle being pulled was also painful but knowing that was the end brought comfort to me.

Cortisone shots are injections that may help relieve pain and inflammation in a specific area of your body. They are commonly injected into joints such as the ankle, elbow, hip, knee, shoulder, spine and wrist. When injected into small joints or tight spaces, they may be much more uncomfortable. Cortisone injections are among the most commonly used treatments in orthopedics. Anti-inflammatory medications can be taken orally, but this distributes the medication in very small doses throughout the entire body. A cortisone injection, on the other hand, places a large, powerful dose directly at the location of the inflammation. Therefore the medication acts very powerfully against the problem. Cortisone is an anti-inflammatory medication, not a pain killer. However, because it reduces inflammation, pain often subsides. Cortisone injections usually work within a few days and the effects can last up to several weeks. My dosage lasted about one week. Then the symptoms gradually re-surfaced. There are potential side effects of a cortisone shot which are not being told.

- Tendon rupture or weakening of tendons
- Facial flushing, mainly in females
- High Blood Sugar – It gets raised temporarily
- Increased pain to injection site
- Change in skin colour especially to those with darker skin.

Surgery is often the treatment along with cortisone shots and other medications. That's where being aware of alternative solutions can be useful.

Chapter 2
Root Causes Of Diseases

We all need one form of healing or another, for there are many who suffer from various illnesses or diseases. Fortunately, there are many cures for our illnesses. There are also many root causes of the disease that plague us. According to Dr. Mark Stengler, some of the root causes are:

- Nutritional deficiencies
- Hormone imbalance
- Genetic abnormalities
- Sensitivities and allergies
- Neurotransmitter imbalances
- Body Structure and alignment
- Digestive imbalance
- Mental, emotional, spiritual factors
- Toxins
- Infections
- Poor diet.

We have to do our part to diligently search and find the paths that suit us best. I have found that the road from pain to power can be helpful if we want to achieve that power.

Before taking any action, ask "Is this action moving me to a more powerful place?" Rather than saying "I can't", say "I won't". Look at things on the bright side. "I should" becomes "I could" and look at life as an adventure. Decide what you want in the situation you are presently in and start to act on it.

Recently, I came across a list of Five Causes of Premature Aging which I found interesting:

1. Free Radical damage to Cells.
    Under normal circumstances, your body's natural anti-oxidants can neutralize harmful free radicals, but system stressors like poor diet and environmental toxins can tip the scales in the favour of oxidation damage.
2. Immune System deterioration.
    As you age, your body produces less immune cells and does a poorer job of quickly getting those cells to the places they're needed. The result? You get sick more often and it takes you longer to recover.
3. Hormone Imbalance
    Hormones are how your brain sends instructions to your organs. As we age three things happen to our bodies. We create less hormones, organs become less responsive to our hormones, or our hormones aren't metabolized from our bloodstream. Like insulin, for example… as we age our cells become less responsive to insulin which can lead to type 2 diabetes.
4. Decreased Organ Function
    Almost every organ in your body becomes less efficient as the cells in them age. Older cells have problems dividing properly and this can lead to deadly cancers.
5. Neurological Deterioration
    One in three seniors die from Alzheimer's or another type of neurodegenerative disease.

Three things to slow down these five causes of premature aging are:

–   stay physically active
–   eat a healthy diet
–   take rejuvenation anti-aging supplement every day.

Chapter 3
Kinds of Healing

There are several types or kinds of healing.

The following are in no particular order of importance, because they are all equally important.

Neither is this list limited to only those mentioned below.

1. Healing by Thought.

Motivational speakers often say "Your thoughts create your life: They create your reality". The road to any kind of success in life starts in the mind. Ninety percent of our thoughts are the same as yesterday. We go over in our minds the same thoughts we thought yesterday. If you are one of those people who wake up in the middle of the night and can't fall asleep, you've probably noticed that you are thinking the same things that you thought of the night before when you woke up in the middle of the night.

Unfortunately, the same thoughts always lead to the same choices.
Those same choices always lead to the same behaviours.
The same behaviours always lead to the same experiences.
The same experiences always create the same emotions.
The same emotions drive us to the same thoughts.

What do we do?

According to Dr. Joe Dispenza, all you have to do is 'Change Your Thoughts'.

That's easy to say. The question is how?

1. Learn Something New.
    Every time you learn something new, you add a new stitch to your brain. Whenever you make your brain work differently, you're changing your mind. Mind is the brain in action. You can change your brain by thinking differently.

    You'll add something different to your brain, so your thoughts won't be the same as yesterday's thoughts. Like learning a new language, doing crossword puzzles, reading, and so on. You start thinking differently. Your thoughts lead to your feelings which causes you to act according to those feelings.

2. Brain Entrainment.
    Brain entrainment is a sound technology that changes your brainwaves and guides your mind into an optimal state for positive transformation, deeper self- awareness and effortless gratitude. According to Brain Specialist Morry Zelcovitch, Brain Entrainment has tremendous positive benefits on your creativity, learning and stress relief, and is one of the many gratitude-boosting technologies you can use daily.

3. Subliminal Audios.
    These are audio tracks laced with subliminal messages that are designed to reprogram your subconscious mind using hundreds of thousands of barely audible positive statements. These subliminal messages are powerful because they penetrate below the level of the conscious mind. The result is profound behavioural change on auto-pilot. Subliminal audios are a great choice if you're busy, because they work in the background. That means that you can be doing chores or even working while listening to them.

4. Daily Gratitude Journal.

    When you start or end your day by writing what you are grateful for in a daily gratitude journal, you are training your mind to be constantly focused on things to be grateful for every minute of every day. Many gratitude enthusiasts recommend writing down five things you're grateful for daily. This number is just enough to get your mind jogging, but not too much that it becomes a chore.

5. Meditation.

    Meditation may not mean the same thing for everyone and there are various ways people meditate. Some sit still or cross-legged and hum or repeat words, while some stand or even meditate while walking. Whichever way one choses to meditate does not matter. The process of meditation helps one to detach from accumulated stress, anxiety and negative charges inside you, so your thoughts and emotions can be more in tune with gratitude.

6. Visualization.

    By consciously visualizing the people, outcomes and situations that you're grateful for, you are training your subconscious mind to feel deeper gratitude for them and you're even allowing more of them into your life. Don't just visualize the positive outcomes you want into your life, but also visualize how you will feel once those outcomes become reality.

7. Affirmations.

    Affirmations are another way to retune your subconscious mind for a more grateful outlook and motivate yourself for success. All you have to do is repeatedly recite a positive statement that aligns with your desired outcome. For instance, if you are concerned about your health, you can say: "I love my body" or "I am healthy" as many times a day as is possible. If you're creating many affirmations, write them down in the present tense. This way you are reassuring your mind that the contents of your affirmation are happening as fact and it will then act accordingly.

The following is a list of affirmations you may choose from:

Everything I do is a success.
There is plenty of resources for everyone, including me.
There are plenty of customers for my services.
I establish a new awareness of success.
I am blessed beyond my fondest dreams.
Divine intelligence gives me all the riches I can use.
Golden opportunities are everywhere for me.

So we've begun to work on our minds. We discover that there are hindrances in our way. We don't understand what these hindrances are, so how can we get them out of our way. We are fully aware that the best time for "New Beginnings" is now, but what are these blocks or hindrances holding us back?

Blocks or Hindrances Holding Us Back

UNFORGIVENESS

We can never be free of bitterness as long as we continue to think unforgiving thoughts. I've heard it said that un-forgiveness can be compared to drinking poison while hoping that the other person will die from it. Simultaneously, the walk of forgiveness has been compared to an onion with many layers. As you deal with the biggest hurts you think you are over it, but then other levels of hurt is being revealed.

At the root of virtually all spiritual practices is the notion of forgiveness. To forgive is to "For-Give" before the other person forgives you. In other words, "Forgive-ness" has to begin with you first. Think about every single person who has ever harmed you, cheated you, defrauded you, or said unkind things about you. Your experience of them is nothing more than a thought that you carry around with you. These thoughts of resentment, anger, and hate represent slow debilitating energies that will disempower you. No matter how justified we feel we are, no matter what 'they' (our mother, our father, our sister or brother) did, if we insist on holding on to the past, then we'll never be free. If we are holding on to the past, we cannot be in the present. It's only in the now or present moment that our thoughts and words are powerful. If we could release them, we would know more peace. That's where repentance comes in. Since un-forgiveness is a heart issue and repentance starts in the heart, that's where the healing must take place. We must decide in our hearts to forgive that person whom we believe has harmed us. The reason we need to change these thoughts is because most of the time, they are detrimental to our own health. In many cases we need to do forgiveness work because of unforgiving thoughts. Thoughts of bitterness can't create joy. We can never be free of bitterness as long as we continue to think unforgiving thoughts.

When we blame someone, we give our own power away because we are placing the responsibility for our feeling on someone else. Taking responsibility for our own feelings and reactions is mastering our ability to respond. We therefore, learn to consciously choose rather than simply react.

Forgiveness is a confusing concept for most of us. That is because we tend to confuse forgiveness for acceptance. Forgiving someone does not mean that we condone their behaviour. The act of forgiveness takes place in our own mind. It has nothing to do with the other person. It has everything to do with us setting ourselves free from the pain. It is simply an act of releasing ourselves from the negative energy that we have chosen to hold on to.

On the other hand, forgiveness doesn't mean allowing the painful behaviours or actions to continue in our lives. In some cases, forgiveness means," letting go." We forgive that person and then release him or her. Then take a stand and set healthy boundaries between him or her and us. This is often a most loving thing to do for ourselves and others as well, as there are usually others who are affected by that act of un-forgiveness.

No matter what our reasons are for having bitter unforgiving feelings, we have a choice. We can choose to stay stuck and resentful thus being in isolation from others or we can do ourselves a favour by willingly forgiving what happened in the past, letting it go and then moving on to a joyous fulfilling life. We have the freedom to make our lives anything we want it to be because we have freedom of choice.

So, choose to forgive. Forgiveness lightens your load, lifts weight off your shoulders and eliminates baggage. You may ask, does forgiving someone make you physically lighter? Your mind says "yes", suggests Ryan Fehr, assistant professor of management at the University of Washington, in an article published in Social Psychology and Personality Science. His findings indicate that the simple act of forgiveness can make hills appear less steep and even allow you to jump higher. In the mind's eye, holding on to anger or resentment is similar to hauling a heavier load up the hill.

So let us try to understand that everyone is doing the best they can at any given moment. People can only do so much with the understanding, awareness, and knowledge that they have.

LACK OF GRATITUDE

It seems next to impossible to read any self-help book these days without coming across advice to "develop an attitude of gratitude." But why? How does feeling grateful help us?

When our lives seem full of troubles, it seems difficult to maintain an Attitude of Gratitude. All we see are our problems, like a dark cloud on a stormy night casting shadows on our lives. The days when things are going smoothly, we often take those 'precious moments' for granted. We get caught up in the bliss comfort and familiarity of it all. We just simply forget to be thankful.

What then is Gratitude?

Gratitude means thankfulness, counting our blessings, noticing simple pleasures, and acknowledging everything that you receive. It means learning to live your life as if everything were a miracle and being aware on a continuous basis of how much we have been given.

Historically, various cultures have taught that expressing gratitude is virtuous. It is considered the greatest virtue, the parent of all the others. Researchers are discovering that there are many positive outcomes to adopting the feeling of gratitude.

The practice has a powerful effect on the psyche with many associated benefits: physical, mental and spiritual. Gratitude shifts your focus from what your life lacks to the abundance that is already present. When the brain feels gratitude, it activates areas responsible for feelings of reward, moral cognition, subjective value judgments, compassion, economic decision making and self-motivation. Grateful people report feeling healthy and tend to experience fewer aches and pains. They are more likely to go see a doctor regularly and take care of their health. Practicing gratitude helps to increase quality of sleep, reduces the time needed to fall asleep and improves sleep duration. Expressions of gratitude promote health and healing for both ourselves and others. Regularly expressing gratitude helps to increase our energy level, reduce stress, boost our immune system, balance our hormones and promote heart health.

How?

Gratitude is a heart-centered approach to being at peace with yourself and with all you have. Gratitude is a habit. It's a way of looking at the world and all the good things in it with a feeling of appreciation for God, regardless of whether or not your present situation is to your liking. Gratitude is an acknowledgment that something of value has been received, recognised and appreciated. Complainers always find that they have little good in their life or they do not enjoy what they do have. Taking time to experience gratitude can make you happier and even healthier. By taking a few moments to write a list of things, big and small that you're thankful for every day, you are placing yourself in position to practice generosity. We all know that giving is a right thing to do. It turns out that generosity also provides some tangible rewards for the giver. So let us open our hearts to those less fortunate, and anyone who has enhanced our lives and offer a token of thanks. This could be in the form of a note, a present, or some other meaningful expression of appreciation.

Gratitude bestows Reverence, allowing us to encounter everyday epiphanies, those transcendent moments of awe that forever change how we experience life and the world. We even want to be grateful for the lessons we have, for those lessons are little packages of treasure that have been given to us. As we learn from them, our lives change for the better. So whether the lesson is a 'problem' that has cropped up or an opportunity to see an old negative pattern within us, that is the time to seize the moment and 'Rejoice' in it.

Gratitude brings more to be grateful about. It increases our abundant life. It lifts up the spirit and can move us from adversity to acceptance if we will allow it. Lack of gratitude or complaining brings little to rejoice about. We only remain stuck in the same pattern of not appreciating.

Gratitude can deepen your spiritual practice. It puts you in touch with your Maker. You come to realize that you are not alone. You don't just exist. You are loved no matter what. Practice being grateful in the good times when there is joy with no struggle as well as the bad when there is lack and struggle. Here are a few gratitude examples to get you started:

I am grateful for what I often take for granted.

I am grateful for a place to live.

I am grateful for the clothes that I have to wear and food to eat.

I am grateful for the beauty that surrounds me. The sun and stars and the seasons that change.

I am grateful for the people in my life, especially those that love me unconditionally.

This is the key to spiritual gratitude that will unlock the door to a happy and fulfilled life. If you have little in your life now, it will increase. If you have an abundant life now, it will also increase.

LACK OF TRUST

This is the least thought about hindrance to our healing. It is like a still small voice; so quiet that it is unheard because we are not trained to listen to it. On the other hand, many people do not trust themselves. This causes chaos in our normal lives. Trust, like anything else comes from repetition.

It is a habit. You learn to trust a result when it repeats again and again. How does one trust? Start with one tiny win. By getting the same result again and again you will soon forget the past. Many people say they cannot enjoy today because of something that happened in the past. Since they did not do something or do it in a certain way in the past, they cannot live a full life today. Because they no longer have something they had in the past, they will not accept love now. They cannot enjoy today. Because something unpleasant happened when they did something once, they are certain it will happen again today. Because they once did something that they are sorry for, they are sure they are bad people forever. Because once someone did something to them, it is now all the other person's fault that their life is not where they want it to be. Because they became angry over a situation in the past they will hold onto that self-righteousness. Because of some very old experience where they were treated badly, they cannot forgive and forget.

STRESS

According to Readers Digest, citing The Mayo Clinic, a nervous breakdown also commonly referred to as a mental or emotional breakdown, is used to describe a situation in which someone cannot function normally because of overwhelming stress. Stress is a normal part of life. It is unavoidable. It is a fear reaction to life and its constant changes. At times it serves us a useful purpose. It can motivate us to get that work done, or run the last mile of a marathon. But if we don't get a handle of stress and it becomes long term it can seriously interfere with our jobs, family life and health. Stress is when your brain and body are not in alignment. Everyone has different triggers because we are all different. Some triggers may be Fear and Uncertainty; Attitudes and Perception; Unrealistic expectations and Change. Sometimes the stress comes from inside, rather than outside. Stress levels will differ based on our personality and how we respond to situations. Some people have the ability to let everything 'roll off their back'. To them, work stresses and life stresses are just minor bumps in the road. Others literally worry themselves sick. Worrying is feeling uneasy or being overly concerned about a situation or problem. With excessive worrying, the mind and body go into over-drive as one constantly focuses on "what might happen". This chronic worry and emotional stress can trigger a host of health problems affecting the digestive system. These lead to difficulty swallowing, dizziness, dry mouth, fast heartbeat, fatigue, headaches, inability to concentrate, irritability, muscle aches, muscle tension, nausea, nervous energy, rapid breathing, shortness of breath, sweating, trembling and twitching, including irritable bowel syndrome. If left untreated, chronic stress causes inflammation by modulating key inflammatory pathways in the body. Although these effects are a response to stress, stress is simply the trigger. Whether or not one becomes ill depends on how one handles stress. What we call stress is simply a fear reaction to life and to the constant change that is inevitable. This fear might just be false evidence that appears real to us. Yet we focus on that evidence as though it is real even before we take the time to check it out. This may sound easy to do, "just take the time to check things out" and you'll eliminate the need for stress in our life. This is a process that most of us struggle with. The fear grips us before we realize it and our emotions quickly kick into high gear with no warning that we are stressing ourselves out. A peaceful, relaxed person (maybe two percent of the population) is seldom frightened or stressed. Some early symptoms of stress are: teeth grinding, apathy or lack of energy, trouble concentrating, bursts of anger, depression. These can slip by unnoticed if we are not aware that we are stressed. So if we feel stressed most of the time, we need to ask ourselves "what are we afraid of." Then acknowledge whatever you think it is. Go a little further and ask yourself whether what we are afraid of is true. In most cases it is not. You then have the power to let it go and not worry about it anymore.

Chapter 4
Healing Visualizations

Healing Visualizations are really healing meditations designed to focus one's attention, promote a positive attitude and change one's beliefs. The crux of visualization therapy is to use the power of the mind to heal the body.

The Power of Emotions.

Emotions are energy in motion and our feelings affect our social life. Every emotion falls into a continuum of intensity for different feeling states. For instance, the state of contentment means that energy is moving at a slower rate, whereas at the state of boredom, there is very little momentum. The emotional energy we bring to each situation has an effect on the outcome we create. So let us try to put more positivity into our lives.

Dr. Masaru Emoto has done extensive experiments using frozen water to prove the power of emotion. He used positive words such as "beautiful", "nice" and "lovely" to create beautiful snowflake-like structures. Since up to sixty percent of our body is comprised of water, he concluded that if our thoughts can do that to water, imagine what our thoughts can do to our bodies. Our thoughts really do change our reality.

Others who used Rice Experiments using positive words like 'I love you', found that the rice remained nice. If they used negative words like 'I hate you', the rice turned brown.

So our negative thoughts can match our reality.

One very dangerous emotion that we all face is Fear.

What is Fear?

Many of us live not just with fear but from fear. We live from fear when we make decisions out of fear. When we live from fear, we don't risk and when we don't risk, we don't grow. That is a high price to pay. If fear is the thief, then the ransom is personal potential.

Fear is and always has been the greatest enemy of mankind. When Franklin D. Roosevelt said, "the only thing we have to fear is fear itself", he was saying that the emotion of fear, rather than the reality of what we fear, is what causes us anxiety, stress and unhappiness. As adults, everything we ever want in life seem to be on the other side of fear. We simply overvalue what we might lose, rather than what we might gain. We fail to realize that any path we're on only becomes clear after we begin the journey. When we develop the habits of courage and unshakeable self-confidence, a whole new world of possibilities open up for us. Fortunately, the habit of courage can be learned just as any other habit is learned through repetition. We need to constantly face and overcome our fears to build up the kind of courage that will enable us to deal with the inevitable ups and downs of life unafraid. Fear is a silent hidden enemy that locks deep in our subconscious mind. We can identify it by the negative thoughts we think and the destructive voices in our head causing us to do the wrong things. This sabotaging pattern can be subtle and sneaky. Sometimes people might be committed to doing something even though they are worried about not having the time or money to do it. But that's not a reason to stop acting on the goal. By acting on our commitments, we open up opportunities, perhaps to some new resource that will make the whole thing feasible. We must be willing to make the commitment down to the marrow in our bones. It is only through this type of dedication and integrity that amazing things will happen, including the fact that wonderful people will emerge to help. Show up fully for what you want even if it takes you into foreign territory. Fear isn't always a bad thing. It's fear, after all that keeps us from straying too close to a ledge or from approaching a wild animal. However, when it comes to pursuing our goals, fear is often the number one thing holding us back. The root source of most fear is childhood conditioning, usually associated with destructive criticism.

There Are Different Kinds Of FEAR.

Some of the most common ones are:

Fear of Failure.

Fear of failure or "atychiphobia" can be so paralyzing that it can prevent us from moving forward to achieve our true goals. People who suffer from this fear often subconsciously undermine their own efforts to avoid disappointment or failure. They think that they can't do and achieve what other people achieve, so they don't even try.

Many people who grow up with overly critical parents carry the humiliation and negativity into adulthood with them. This fear can show up as a reluctant to try something new, self-sabotage, anxiety, low self-esteem and perfectionism. When taken to the extreme, we become totally preoccupied with not making a mistake which leads to perfectionism and with constantly seeking approval for security's sake. They are unable to achieve a work-life balance and never feel happy no matter how much money they acquire.

This fear we feel when faced with a major life change is closely connected with shame. The sense that there is something basically flawed inside that might cause us to fail and to be seen by others as a failure, can immobilize us before we begin. Many people organize their lives around never having to feel that, and one of the best ways to avoid the shameful feeling of failure is to avoid the risk of a new enterprise, says Burgo. Some people with a fear of failure may appear successful in one area such as wealth accumulation but suffer in their interpersonal relationships. They are unable to achieve a work-life balance and never feel happy no matter how much money they acquire.

Fear of failure is the single greatest obstacle to success in adult life. We're afraid we won't succeed if we try something new. We fear that we will never "make it" doing what we are passionate about so we allow our dreams to float away from us.

Fear of failure keeps many of us from taking risks, thus binding us to a life of complacency. Risks are often necessary and complacency is the enemy of success. Instead of allowing our fear to hold us back, it is important to turn that fear into fuel to get us going. It is not easy to overcome the fear of failure, but once we build up the confidence to not let it hold us back we can achieve much more. Ask what it is that we're afraid of and then take actions to negate that fear. If we are able to recognize the fears and overcome them, we can then turn our fears into a powerful motivator rather than a shackle that binds us.

Fear of Rejection.

Fear of rejection is a deep-seated human fear that can be especially problematic. Humans long to be accepted and this basic primitive need is entrenched in our very survival as a species.

Fear of rejection, embarrassment and or ridiculed are directly tied to our self-esteem. It activates an unconscious protection mechanism in the brain anytime we feel that we may experience emotional or physical pain. Whether we realize it or not, this fear lurks deep in the mind and begin taking shape in childhood. As children, when we did what pleased our parents, teachers or authority figures, they gave us love and approval. However, when we did things they did not like, they withdrew their love and approval, which we interpreted as rejection. Over the years, this fear continues to brew inside us causing us to avoid risks and rejecting opportunities presented to us to ironically protect us from rejection itself. As a result, we develop an "I can't" attitude. We feel the fear in the front of the body, the stomach, moving upwards causing the heart to beat rapidly and our breathing heavily as if we've just run a marathon. This kind of fear interferes with performance and inhibits expression. We become paralyzed when it's time to take action. Children who grow up in dysfunctional families may go to unhealthy extremes to be accepted by peers and later by romantic partners. They usually suffer from low self-esteem and fear being ostracized or rejected.

They imagine catastrophic consequences as a result of not fitting in. On the other hand, if they become or go overboard they may inadvertently cause the rejection which they struggle so hard to avoid.

The only way out is to stop disguising fear with denial or "playing it safe" and confront it head on. When we force ourselves to face the fear of rejection, our self-esteem goes up, our self-respect increases and our sense of personal pride grows.

The opposite of fear is actually love, self-love, and self-respect. Acting with courage in a fearful situation is a simple technique that boosts regard for ourselves to such a degree that our fears subside and lose their ability to affect our behaviour and our decisions.

Fear of Change.

Change is inevitable. It is something that is inescapable in the life of any organization; a political organization not excluded, is change and transition. Sometimes the change takes a while and sometimes, out if necessity it comes a bit more rapidly but one way or the other change comes. Change is usually what we want the other person to do, isn't it? When we speak about the other person, we want to include the government, big business, the boss or co-worker, the Internal Revenue Service, foreigners, the school, husband, wife, mother, father, the children, etcetra, anyone other than ourselves. We don't want to change, but we want everybody else to change so our lives will be different. Yet, any changes that we are going to make at all have to come from within ourselves.

Change means that we free ourselves from feelings of isolation, separation, loneliness, anger, fear and pain. We create lives filled with wonderful peacefulness, where we can relax and enjoy life as it comes to us-where we know that everything will be all right.

Fear of change or changing things is called Metathesiophobia. It is often linked with Tropophobia, which is the fear of moving. Fear isn't something to deal with and get past. It may mean the moment is near, you need to take action now, because it signals that a window of opportunity has opened in front of you. That part of you that has gone through this in the past knows and is changing and begging you to pay attention and put your body on full alert. This means that getting past the fears and just "doing it" is more important than ever. If we're making an unconventional change for example, downshifting a job to claim more free time or moving to a smaller house to save money, you may worry that others will see you as an odd-ball or slacker, or in some other way judge you as being 'wrong'. Again, getting past our fears is doing what we "must do."

Many of us think that fear is a sign of danger, that if we feel any kind of fear it must mean something bad is about to happen and we should try to avoid it. This might have served us well when we were kids, but we are no longer kids. There is a difference between the fear of the unknown that comes from venturing into new territory and the instinctual gut feeling that something isn't right. If you ask yourself which one you are feeling, you will certainly be able to tell.

The thought of making a life change can be so intimidating that even though you want to be a better person, you end up doing nothing, or settling for less than you deserve simply because you are so afraid of that change. It is easier to fail than to succeed.

We need to break through the wall in every area of our lives. We should try to remember that "Life is wonderful." It can be wonderful if we try to enjoy the situations and circumstances that come our way. Set goals and take full responsibility of your life.

Fear of the Unknown.

When you are new to something, like starting a business, learning a new trade or anything unfamiliar to you, there is an extreme amount of insecurity and need to make things perfect. Being perfect removes the likelihood of criticism and increases the likelihood of approval. Not meeting someone's personal standard of perfection does not mean that the result isn't exceptional. More importantly, trying to achieve perfection is often just another way to avoid making a commitment to act.

Your mind fears the unknown because it considers what is known to be far safer. You might not like it but at least it is familiar and you know what to expect. As for the unknowing, your imagination will come up with dozens of potential things to fear about that. And it's all done 'to keep you safe'. Once you know this, then it's easier to understand why you are suddenly coming up with all these fear thoughts. With this knowledge, you will be able to notice when you have these fear thoughts, understand why they are happening and be able to process them so you can let them go. For example, when you hear yourself say, "You will fail. It will be a disaster. You'll get hurt," know that your safety guy is hard at work trying to keep you safe. As soon as you realize this, you won't keep thinking about the thoughts and believing them because you know it is your safety mechanism trying to protect you, which you can now override. You can then start thinking about the positives that may happen if you make this life change. You can start to focus on the good that will come instead of what "might" happen.

Fear of Success.

A common reason people fear success is related to mix messages society sends regarding those who succeed. It has been linked with negative characteristics such as competition, envy or evil. Still others may have internalized verbal abuse such as being told they were losers or would never amount to much. Subsequently, they live down to these expectations.

You may worry about how success in your new endeavor will change your life, your friendship and your feelings about yourself, especially if growing up you picked up the idea that it is dangerous to stand out or be special in any way. If you succeed in becoming the 'new person' you want to be, will old friends abandon you, judge you or envy you?

If you are prone with a certain amount of envy or resentment of those who are more successful than you are, you may be particularly unsettled by the prospect of becoming a target of envy or resentment yourself, says Burgo. This fear often times lead to self-judgment, where you interpret your fear as weakness or a lack of courage. You may tell yourself, "what's wrong with me that I can't move forward?"

Keeping our goal in mind and focusing on that goal will help overcome many of our fears. Then develop a plan and process to achieve that goal. Achieving any goal in life is like swimming with the current. You can't always control it. Trying to do so only creates anxiety. To help with these anxieties, surround yourself with people who believe in you. They can help clarify and direct you towards your goal. Have faith in yourself and trust the process.

Fear of Death.

Fear of death or dying known as thanatophobia, is an abnormal and persistent fear of one's own mortality, which causes severe anxiety and distress.

Though this fear is mostly an unconscious reaction, we may hesitate before big changes because in Burgo's words, "they tend to make us aware of the passage of time in ways that are kind of unpleasant. They bring up ideas about finality and death." When we're stuck in a familiar routine, we lose track of the passage of time, but the big markers in our lives really bring into consciousness the fact that our lives are moving toward their end. That's uncomfortable.

Other Common Fears are:

The Fear of Commitment or Intimacy. This fear closely resembles the fear of not being loved.

You may want approval of your mom or dad (even if you're over forty);

You may want approval of your partner or spouse;

You may want approval of your family members;

You may want approval of your friends (maybe your face book friends you may not even know).

This fear of not being loved or not being good enough, stops us from becoming "Great". It stops us from playing big and making a true impact in this world. It sabotages success whenever we see any type of it. The only person we need to have approval of is ourselves. Everyone else's approval has nothing to do with us and everything to do with them. We cannot control how they feel, we can only control how we feel.

According to surveys done in the U.S. approximately seventeen percent of adults suffer from a fear of intimacy or closeness in relationships.

Fear of Spiders (arachnophobia) is an intense and irrational fear of spiders.

Fear of Flying.

A fear of flying is the fear of being on board a helicopter or airplane while it is flying in the air above the ground.

Fear of Heights.

Acrophobia is an irrational fear of heights. This fear has its roots as a healthy defense to keep us safe from doing dangerous things such as "walking off a cliff."

Fear of Public Speaking.

Fear of public speaking (glossophobia) can afflict people of all walks of life. Well known speakers confess that they feel fear before they get on stage. They have learned to just push past the fear.

Fear of the Dark.

This irrational fear is common in millions of young children whose anxiety is heightened when the lights go out at bedtime.

Truths about Fear.

Fear will not go away as long as you continue to grow.

The only way to get rid of fear is to go out and do it. Face it head on. The "doing it" comes before the feeling of feeling better about yourself. You can expect to feel fear whenever you are on unfamiliar territory – but so does everybody else. Fear is a signal to move ahead – not retreat, if you want to grow.

Fear and Anger are present in all diseases. Their role is to suppress the immune system in the body. This is because negative emotions, such as fear and anger, when held too long create chemical reactions in your body that do not support your health. Fear and anger show up in us as: impatience, irritation, frustration, criticism, judgement, resentment, jealousy, bitterness, muscle tension, jaw pain, anxiety, worry and doubt.

Chapter 5
Healing with Nutrition

Have you heard of healing with nutrition? Nowadays, many people have heard of healing your body with nutritious foods. Back in 2014, I had never heard of that. Yet it is true and definitely was then. Just google "healing with food". I was amazed to see the numerous amount of information there is on that subject. Lack of information from the experts we trust with our lives play a major part of our ignorance on the subject. Our physicians, whom we trust with the health of our bodies, did not focus on nutrition in medical school. However, there are advocates, such as Dr. Josh Axe, DNM, DC, a certified doctor of natural medicine, doctor of chiropractic and clinical nutritionist with a passion to help people get healthy using food as medicine, wrote about how he used nutrition to cure his mother's breast cancer. Another pioneer of nutritional healing is Dr. Max Gerson M.D. 1905 – 1959. Even if many people do not know his name, his impact on the world is monumental. The Gerson Therapy as it is known consists mainly of organic plant-based foods, raw juices each day, coffee enemas, beef liver and natural supplements. Countless thousands have been healed using these nutritional principles, basically alternative methods to treating cancer, pioneered by Dr. Gerson. A Cancer Therapy: Results of Fifty Cases and the Cure of Advanced Cancer by Diet Therapy are Dr. Gerson's most popular books. Several other nutritional books such as Beating Cancer with Nutrition by Dr. Patrick Quillin are readily available.

Many disturbances to our body's natural capabilities can promote diseases. The most popular ones like cancer, heart attack, stroke, diabetes, high blood pressure and low blood pressure can all be treated and healed. We hold the power to unleash our natural healing capabilities by committing to various diets.

One such diet is the Ketogenic Diet, or keto diet for short.

The dictionary describes keto diet as a metabolic state characterized by raised levels of ketone bodies in the body tissues, which is typically pathological in conditions such as diabetes, or may be the consequence of a diet that is very low in carbohydrates.

The Ketogenic diet is not only low in carbohydrates but also high in food fats and proteins. This kind of diet reduces the risk of mutations that occur in the cells along with the free radicals, both of which are causes of colon, lung and breast cancer. Ketosis describes a condition where fat stores are broken down to produce energy, which also produces ketones, a type of acid. The ketogenic diet reduces symptoms in patients with metabolic conditions because it lowers the energy generated from the breakdown of glucose found in simple and complex carbohydrates. Cancer cells thrive off of the energy created from glucose fermentation. The National Institute of Health states that the keto diet shows promise for treating Alzheimer's, Parkinson's, Epilepsy, Autism, Depression, Migraines and Cancer. Some people try to follow a ketogenic low-carb diet in an effort to lose weight and improve their health. When followed correctly, beginning with a brief fast, allowing our bodies to quickly burn through the carbs that are in our system and turn it to fat for fuel. This low carb, high fat diet will raise blood ketone levels. Keytones are a special type of fat that can stimulate the pathways that enhance the growth of new neural networks in the brain. Keytones increase glutathione, a powerful brain protective antioxidant. These keytones provide a new fuel source for your cells and cause most of the unique health benefits of this diet. On a keto diet, your body undergoes many biological adaptations, including a reduction in insulin and increased fat breakdown. When this happens, your liver starts producing large amounts of ketones to supply energy for your brain.

In diabetic patients, ketosis can occur due to the body not having enough insulin to process the glucose in the body. The presence of ketones in the urine is an indicator that a patient's diabetes is not being controlled properly.

The keto diet could have a healthful effect on serious health conditions such as:

- cardiovascular disease
- diabetes
- metabolic syndrome

It may also improve levels of HDL cholesterol also known as "good cholesterol" better than other moderate carbohydrate diets. These health benefits could be due to the loss of excess weight and eating of healthier foods rather than a reduction in carbohydrates.

According to Miriam Kalamian, EdM, MS,CNS., a nutrition educator and consultant specializing in the implementation of ketogenic therapies, "To reach ketosis, you'll be eliminating a lot of the foods that are staples in your current diet. Out goes sugar in any of its forms, both obvious in cookies and sneaky in canned tomato sauce. Inflammatory grains: wheat, corn and oats. Starchy vegetables like potatoes, also sweet potatoes, cooked carrots. The list also includes dairy fats like butter, ghee, heavy cream and some dairy products such as milk are out. Hard cheese in small amounts are ok."

Examples of ketogenic approved foods include: pastured beef and dairy products (including eggs), organic poultry, wild fish and seafood. Vegetables and fruits low in carbohydrates (including cabbage, asparagus, lemons and limes), healthy fats such as avocados and coconut oil, along with almonds, walnuts and seeds are usually permitted.

Committing to a ketogenic diet can delay the development of tumors and increase the survival rate for patients by greater than fifty percent.

BETA GLUCANS.

Beta Glucan is one of the most balancing immune boosters in the body. It is often referred to as a 'bio logical response modifier' which helps to bind to white blood cells and improve their immune coordination.

Beta glucans are naturally-occurring compounds found in foods, but not in the human body. These complex sugar molecules supplement the immune system in order to design well targeted attacks on cancer and other foreign agents in the body. Beta glucans provide immunomodulation and treat excessive inflammation due to autoimmune responses.

Beta glucans protect the body from various diseases by activating immune cells such as antibodies natural killer cells, cytokines, T-cells and macrophages. Together these cells coordinate attacks on tumor growth.

Beta glucan supplementation has been shown in research to lower the rate of cancer cell concentration by effectively detecting and destroying their targets.

Some common foods which contain beta glucans are yeast, mushrooms, fermented foods, certain algae and indigestible soluble fibres including oats and barley. The hearty health soluble fibre in oatmeal has been shown to lower cholesterol in the body. Soluble fibre can also be found in beans, lentils, peas and fruit. We need these essential additions to our diet.

JUICING

Juicing is an amazing tool which anyone can use to decrease the likelihood of developing most diseases. It is a powerful and simple way to boost your antioxidant levels and promote your body's ability to prevent, fight and heal from many diseases including cancer. Juicing cruciferous vegetable sprouts such as kale, broccoli and cauliflower inundates the body with powerful antioxidants and cancer fighting tools to boost the immune system and improve health. In fact, juicing some vegetables and fruit can supply a higher amount of nutrients for absorption in comparison to eating the entire raw or cooked food source on its own. To receive the greatest benefits with minimal effort, try juicing cruciferous vegetables since they contain phytochemicals which have profound anti-aging, anti-cancer and antioxidant properties. Kale, broccoli and cauliflower sprouts are only required in small concentrations to reap health benefits. Such sprouts provide natural enzymes for the body to fight cancer by reducing free radicals and inflammation. Many practitioners recommend cancer patients consume 32 to 64 ounces of fresh green juices each day to help slow cancer growth. For prevention, eight to 16 ounces can be a great strategy to ensure your body is receiving sufficient micronutrients.

FERMENTED FOODS.

Fermented foods are good for a healthy gut. There are trillions of tiny creatures living in our bodies. These good bacteria, particularly those in our gut, may improve digestion, boost immunity and may even help us get leaner. Thanks to a product of fermentation called Acetylcholine, which helps stimulate the movement of food through the intestine. It improves blood circulation, prevents constipation and helps crank up gastric juices when they are insufficient and down and regulates them when there is too much. Eating foods packed with probiotics – good bacteria that live in your gut is one way to boost up your gut health. Excellent sources for healthy bacteria are fermented foods also referred to as cultured foods, and beverages. Bacteroidetes are a main type of bacteria found in fermented foods which produce a substance known as butyrate. Butyrate possesses its own cancer fighting properties and is involved in enzymatic processes associated with breaking down starch. A healthy gut microbiota is important in regulating the entire health of the whole body and mind.

Those at increased risk for metabolic conditions and cancer typically have elevated concentrations of harmful bacteria in their gut microbiomes. Some cancers associated with unhealthy gut bacteria are colorectal cancer, pancreatic carcinoma and gallbladder cancer.

For people coping with diabetes, fermented foods make no demands on the pancreas because sugars are already broken down.

Adding fermented dairy products such as yogurt and kefir with live cultures from grass-fed cows to your diet is an added benefit to your healing. Other cultured foods and vegetables are: Kombucha, a tangy, effervescent tea (black or green)

Sauerkraut, just cabbage and salt
Miso, paste made from barley, rice or soybeans
Tempeh, naturally fermented soybeans
Kimchi, sauerkraut's Korean cousin (spicy cabbage)

and other fermented foods and beverages are also sources of good bacteria.

Raw, cultured vegetables could be considered pickled because of the addition of Celtic sea salt, but it is not a term general used. This is because someone might think that they have vinegar in them, and they do not.

Many practitioners recommend two to four servings of fermented foods each day to improve health and prevent or slow cancer growth.

Note of caution: Take things slow when first adding fermented foods to your diet to avoid painful gas and bloating.

VITAMIN D.

An important component to the central nervous system and the health of the entire body is Vitamin D. This vital nutrient has anti-inflammatory and antioxidant abilities which continue to astound researchers. Studies find that vitamin D is associated with reducing autoimmune complications and can limit the release of natural killer cell secretions when situations are unwarranted such as during pregnancy.

One of the key functions of vitamin D is its ability to balance the inflammatory pathways linked to cancer and promote the production of proteins such as GcMAF which regulates cancer cells. GcMAF (or Gc protein-derived macrophage activating factor) is a protein produced by modification of Vitamin D-binding protein. Biochemically, GcMAF results from sequential deglycosylation of the vitamin D-binding protein which is naturally promoted by B and T cells.

GcMAF requires vitamin D in order to be created and fulfill its vital functions to maintaining the health of all cells and tissues. GcMAF has been shown to reverse breast cancer by preventing cancer cells from multiplying. Vitamin D therapy therefore also promotes GcMAF function and the ability to treat lymphoma, bladder, ovarian and head and neck cancers among many others.

Dr. Jeff Bradstreet presented findings of treating more than 11,000 patients with various chronic illnesses using GcMAF therapy. He had eighty five percent success rate, with fifteen percent seeing the full remission of their illness. Without Vitamin D, GcMAF cannot be produced because GcMAF contains binding proteins and cellular receptors requiring Vitamin D activation.

Physicians rarely check your vitamin D levels during your regular annual physical checkups unless you specifically ask them to do so. If a child is diagnosed with autism, it would be wise to have their Vitamin D level checked.

There is a common misnomer that we can get enough vitamin D3 just from the foods we eat and from the sun. However, large scale studies find that deficiency is widespread in both adults and children. Maybe it is because there are not very many naturally occurring dietary sources of vitamin D. According to the American Journal of Public Health, supplementation could reduce cancer incidence and mortality at low cost with few or no adverse effects. It can be found in oily fish like salmon, mackerel, and tuna, as well as in fish liver oils.

ENZYMES.

Your body contains numerous enzymes required for performing normal physiological processes. An enzyme can no longer serve its function when certain conditions are not met. Instead they become unraveled. Enzymes promote anti-inflammatory effects, stimulate anti-cancer substances and assist in the removal of toxins from the body.

It is very important that the proper balance of pH in our bodies is met. Unfortunately, our diets often leave our internal organs swamped in an environment full of excess acidity and affect the ability of enzymes to perform. The toxins in the air we breathe, the water we drink, the personal care and household cleaning products we use and many other lifestyle conditions further exacerbate this problem which can lead to diseases.

We must consciously choose to replenish the enzymes in our body and promote a stable environment for them to function. Enzymes are found in foods such as raw fruits and vegetables, fermented vegetables and legumes. Citrus fruits such as lemons and limes are rich in organic acids which help to lower the acidity in our bodies and improve natural functions

TUMERIC.

Tumeric is a spice which you can add to your favourite curry dishes, Indian cuisines and traditional soups and stews. It is excellent mixed in with healthy fats such as pastured milk. Research in clinical studies has shown that curcumin found in turmeric root has powerful abilities to treat cancer symptoms, including its ability to fight inflammation.

A promising study published in Neurology Research International titled "The Potential of curcumin in treatment of Spinal Cord Injury," suggests that the ancient Indian spice, turmeric, and its primary polyphenol curcumin, may provide victims of spinal cord injury a safer and more effective approach than conventional treatment which relies primarily on surgery and corticosteroids, a class of anti-inflammatory drugs notorious for adverse health effects. Curcumin has been validated in hundreds of studies to have immense value in treating a wide range of inflammatory based diseases.

Tumeric exhibits the same inflammation prevention control as do synthetic anti-inflammatory drugs like Tylenol and is supported by more than 570 studies. What is unique about turmeric is that it combats inflammation through both the mechanisms simultaneously: They neutralize inflammation causing free radicals in the body with a flood of antioxidants or they stop the body from producing the chemicals that initiate inflammation in the first place. This is how aspirin and over the counter pain meds work. Tumeric contains the polyphenol curcumin, which has been found to be useful in reducing cancer risk. Curcumin seems to be able to kill cancer cells and prevent more from growing. Curcumin may also be able to destroy multi-drug resistant cancer and cancer stem cells and also protect against radiation induced damage according to The Food Revolution Network, Inc. Tumeric has been proven to reduce or eliminate pain better than some healing prescription medications. A 2004 study published in the journal Oncogene found that components of turmeric were effective alternatives to the drugs aspirin, ibuprofen, sunlindac, naproxen and diclofenac, to name a few. The reason is because turmeric doesn't just fight pain and inflammation, it does so much more. Its multi-pronged approach allows it to work wonders for aches, pain and arthritis by stopping inflammation at the source, while also strongly supporting the immune system with antioxidants.

Curcumin promotes the production of other antioxidant compounds such as glutathione and prevents oxidative damage or stress done to organs, thereby supporting joint and bone health. It is said to enhance cognitive function, boosts immune response and promote body detoxification. Since nearly all diseases and ailments can be traced back to inflammation and oxidative stress, it seem like there's almost nothing that turmeric cannot heal.

Curcumin should be mixed with peperine from black pepper and taken with a fat-based meal for optimal absorption.

DETOXIFICATION.

Detoxification is a requirement in the process of healing the body and treating symptoms of all the major diseases.

Various detoxification pathways can become blocked or underused which leads to a buildup of carcinogens and the formation of cancer and other diseases. Increase healing in your body by removing toxins using any or all of the following detoxification strategies.

Exercise – Increases oxygen flow and opens up pores for detox

Fasting – preferably intermittent fasting, gives the body time to use any glycogen and begin burning stored body fat

Infrared saunas – Stimulates deep tissue for the release of carcinogens

Coffee enemas – Removes toxins along the gastrointestinal tract and can also improve mood

Castor oil packs – Stimulates the flow of toxins out of organs and the intestines

Dry brushing – Stimulates lymphatic flow and glandular function

Consume an anti-cancer diet – decreases toxic burden and decreases inflammation

Drink lemon or mineralizing water – Balances the body's natural pH

Receiving a massage coupled with aromatherapy oils is another excellent technique to

Improve lymphatic function and promote detoxification. Essential oils can boost health in cancer patients and reduce stress and anxiety.

SUNLIGHT

Getting outside in sunlight is beneficial for improving both mental and physical health. Sunlight can improve your mood, create optimism and better support your immune – system's ability to fight off foreign invaders and cancerous cells.

Removing toxins from your body in order to treat diseases is dependent on the proper functioning of your glands. Part of Dr. Johanna Budwig's protocol is to receive naturally-sourced photons from the sun. This creates a magnetic field which attracts electrons into the cells of your body. Dr. Budwig also believed that the sun's rays stimulate the function of glandular organs including the pancreas, salivary glands, bladder, liver and gall bladder. Stimulating energy into your cells is not only vital to heal cancer but can improve the health of your mind as well.

The Budwig Diet

Dr. Budwig was a world leading expert of her time in the 1950's. Her research on fats and their impacts in human microbiology shows that the right combination of quack or cottage cheese (saturated fats) and flaxseed oil (unsaturated fats) has therapeutic properties in preventing, treating, and even curing certain cancers. It was observed that cancer patients had improved oxygen supply to their cells and found relief from all forms and stages of cancer including cancers of the gastrointestinal tract, brain, breast and skin cancers. While researching the pathogenesis of disease and illness as a biochemist in Germany, Dr. Budwig observed that quack contained the very same sulphydryl groups found in cancer treatment drugs. The basic rule with the Budwig diet is "if God made it, then it's fine and try to eat it in the same form that God made it."

ESSENTIAL OILS

Use of Essential Oils are becoming quite popular. The aromatherapy can be combined with massage and other treatments to help address virtually every side effect a cancer patient may be experiencing. It has been said that essential oils can help prevent and treat cancer at the cellular level. Essential oil therapy for cancer is still experimental. However there are many testimonials from people who say that essential oils cured them of cancer.

STRESS RELIEF

Next to sugar consumption, stress is arguably the number one cause of disease in the human body.

One action that all cancer survivors have in common is maintaining a positive attitude and the will to survive. It is a key ingredient for anyone struggling with an illness or disease. In order to keep stress under control, we must accept that there are events that we cannot control. That's why we turn to prayer. By praying, we acknowledge that some situations are beyond us. We need help from a higher source. Join a prayer group.

There are specific techniques in relaxation. Be it meditation or stress management.

Finding the right counselor that resonates with you have been proven to be helpful. Education sessions specific to your situation can help clarify any misunderstanding. Exercise to raise endorphins and increase circulation and cognitive function. Eat healthy well balanced meals. Get enough rest and sleep. Your body needs time to recover from daily stressful events. Learn to say NO to requests that create excessive stress in your life.

Last but not least, spend more time with those you enjoy.

Chapter 6
Holistic Healing

By holistic, I am referring to the use of various instruments to achieve your healing. Thus using medicine, foods, thoughts, faith, etc. I believe that healing comes in various forms and ways, so I do not depend on just one mode or method to obtain my healing.

The ultimate goal of holistic healing is wholeness. To achieve wholeness, we must consider all aspects of our lives including your body, your relationship, your environment, others and your life purpose.

There are three general types of health: physical, mental and spiritual. It is only when we view ourselves from a holistic perspective that we realize that health is really an overall state of being. We are either balanced or unbalanced. The body, mind and soul work as a system with each part contributing equally to the whole person.

What then is holistic healing?

Holistic healing is about bringing any imbalance into alignment with its natural state of functioning. Every organ in our body has a natural or healthy state of functioning as do our emotional, mental and spiritual states. When we are out of balance, we feel like something is out of place. It could be in the form of emotional or physical pain or discord and we naturally want to return to our natural state of harmony where everything works as intended. This process of rebalancing is what is known as holistic healing. This holistic healing bypasses the conventional medical approach. It looks beyond a person's physical state and sees the whole view of their state of

Mary Abdool-Warner

being. It acknowledges that the root cause of a physical illness may be in fact non-physical. For example, holistic healing works when we approach life from all aspects of being.

Physical: Good nutrition, exercise to tone up the body through movement, alignment and awareness, and healthy environment.

Emotional: Release past hurts, forgive. Balance your emotional patterns and behaviours.

Mental: New perspective, positive attitude and goal setting. Using your mind to focus on what you want to accomplish.

Spiritual: Soul purpose, intuitive guidance and divine communication. Listen to your Soul's guidance.

A holistic approach is considered more effective because change occurs on all levels and as a result, positive changes are more likely to last long-term and improve a person's overall quality of life. I personally like the naturopathic route to healing because it is holistic in its approach. It employs various natural means of treating symptoms and the root causes of symptoms. Naturopathic medicine is holistic care. It connects the physical, mental and emotional aspects of the body to find the root cause of disease and its symptoms and treat them using natural and safe methods such as botanical/herbal medicines, acupuncture, homeopathy, dietary and lifestyle modifications, vitamin/mineral supplements and other tools as necessary. The role of the naturopathic physician is to understand and aid the body's efforts to heal from within.

Every one of us sooner or later will walk through hell. It may come through being hurt by some-one, or by hurting some-one. It may come through the battle of cancer not knowing whether this will be the last year on this earth or losing a loved one through cancer. It may be the betrayal of a loved one or going through a divorce. The point is not to give up hope. There is a real and profound power in the suffering we endure if we transform that suffering into a more authentic meaningful life.

Chapter 7
Spiritual Healing

There are various meanings for the term "Spiritual Healing". When I first heard this term, my mind automatically came up with thoughts of heaven, God, angels, miracles and so on. However, when I checked further, I was amazed to discover that this term can also include Spiritual Healing based on science. One profound teacher of this science is Deborah Wayne, founder of the Biofield Healing Institute, Healing with Deborah.com. Deborah testifies that anyone can be healed through her Biofield Healing techniques. She says that your answers are within you and everything is energy.

We should realize that the symptoms we experience are not the root cause of our problems. Our predominant thoughts and feelings are the subtle forms of negative energy which eventually affect our body. So in order to heal, we have to feel by getting in touch with our emotions before they get buried so deep that depression gets a chance to settle in our lives. We can learn how the body speaks by tuning in to our emotions, as emotions cause disease in specific organs. For example, the emotion fear is processed through the kidneys, bladder and reproductive organs which can lead to cancer of the ovaries, prostate, uterine and adrenals. The emotion of anger affects the gall bladder and liver. Stress and worry affect the stomach, pancreas and spleen. Grief and sadness affect the lungs and colon while fight or flight affects the heart and central nervous system. Many may not know that hard-heartedness eventually leads to multiple sclerosis and traumatic events not handled properly can lead to breast cancer. The body tells the story of what's going on in the mind. Therefore, we must immediately explore the feelings we feel to deal with them early rather than later.

Mary Abdool-Warner

Another form of Spiritual Healing which I follow closely is looking to the Maker of the Universe who made everything. There is power in prayer. Through the centuries, prayer and meditation have been used in different forms in different cultures. The prayer can be for someone else or for yourself. Blind studies have shown that when patients are prayed for, there was significant improvement. They experienced a feeling of well -being. Several cancer survivors share their healing stories freely for all to hear and learn from their pain and trials. On thetruthforcancer.com, author and cofounder Ty and Charlene Bollinger have posted several videos of victorious testimonials. One such survivor is Chris Wark, (chrisbeatcancer.com). Chris was diagnosed with stage 4 colon cancer. He used a combination of diet and lifestyle changes plus faith to heal the cancer. Now he is spreading the word and the techniques he used, to all who will listen. He interviews cases of those who went through and those going through similar circumstances as he and boldly shares those testimonies with the world. I have deliberately left out the last names of the survivors for various reasons.

One such testimony is that of Ed, who was diagnosed with stage three C prostate cancer in 2008 and is alive today. He followed a similar protocol to Chris and is alive today.

Joanne was diagnosed with brain, bladder and lung cancer. She too, followed a similar protocol and is a healthy woman today. Susan was diagnosed with stage four ovarian cancer in 2016. She followed a vegan diet and is now cancer free. Norma was diagnosed with breast cancer in 2016. She followed a paleo diet and is now healthy. Angela and Gerald husband and wife were diagnosed with brain tumor and melanoma in 1994. Their positive attitude and change of diet helped them survive. There are many more remarkable testimonies posted on his website. Beating cancer God's way is not a promise for a 'cure'. It is a lifestyle approach designed to help people regain control of their lives. It is filled with spiritual inspiration, easy to follow nutrition guidelines, basic supplement and essential oil user tips and resources to help the normal cancer patient revisit their health and experience an abundant life. Sometimes "beating cancer," is when someone finds emotional peace or mental stability during their crisis. Other times "beating cancer" is when someone starts to sleep better, their pain goes away or their desire to live returns. For others, "beating cancer" is when someone wins the battle and ends up cancer free.

Several other healing testimonies attribute their healing strictly through faith and prayer. This is the method I used in 2017 while suffering with excruciating pain in my left wrist and hand for several years. At that time, I had not done any research about pain, so I knew nothing about the various modes of healing except for prayer. It took several weeks to be completely pain free, but the pain became less severe with each passing day after I incorporated prayer. I followed Andrew Wommack's Ministries which teaches prayer and faith in God to heal any type of disease. Information and testimonials can be found on Andrew Wommack's website: http:// AWMI.net. Or AWMC.CA

Chapter 8
Be Aware of who is Funding
our Health Campaigns

We should be aware of who is funding breast cancer campaigns. October is Breast Cancer Awareness Month, a time when groups ramp up their advocacy and breast cancer stories fill the media. Every October, I wonder. Will this year's awareness and funds raised mean better health for breast cancer patients? In 1999, The Canadian Breast Cancer Network (CBCN) formed its first partnership with a pharmaceutical company and launched a campaign to raise awareness of anemia in breast cancer patients – a condition the company partner happened to have a drug to treat. That drug turned out to promote tumour growth; in a clinical trial, breast cancer patients given Eprex died sooner than those given a placebo.

In one case, The Food and Drug Administration approved the drug Avastin for breast cancer based on early research and patient demand, only to revoke approval in 2011 after determining the drug was ineffective for breast cancer and posed life-threatening risks. The main beneficiaries of drug access campaigns are pharmaceutical companies, which almost always sponsor them, although the support is seldom obvious.

The price of new cancer drugs has spiralled to six figures for treatments that, at best, may extend life by a few months. As Sharon Batt, an independent scholar, activist and author wrote in her book: Health Advocacy Inc., We need to raise awareness about the practice of drug companies funding campaigns like the CBCN's.

Here is a juicy piece of news that some people may never hear about. The Saturday March 10, 2018, Toronto Star newspaper printed an article 'Pharma bro' gets seven years in prison. "Notorious pharmaceutical exec takes blame after being found guilty of defrauding investors". The article is about a self promoting pharmaceutical executive notorious for trolling critics online, being convicted in a securities fraud case last year. This executive confessed to a U.S. District Judge that he made many mistakes and apologized to investors. He said that he hopes to make amends and learn from his mistakes and apologized to his investors. Many such happenings occur quite frequently.

The take-away from this is for us Consumers to be aware, knowledgeable and accountable for our health. We can no longer rely on the government and their advocates to keep us safe and healthy.

Chapter 9
The Years are Slipping By

I realize that the years are slipping by. I hear other people say "where did the time go?"

So I know that I am not the only one facing this dilemma.

That means that the years are slipping by quickly. By the time one reaches the age of forty, a certain realization hits the mind. Questions start flowing through the mind like a river flowing downstream after a rainy day.

The question is, 'are we happy?' Are we doing what we were put on this earth to do?

What will we be remembered for after we have left this earth?

What kind of legacy are we leaving behind?

It has been said that happiness lengthens our lives. Generally, unhappy people (not their fault) are more likely to develop chronic diseases, cutting their life short. Tragedies happen to us all.

Some people handle trials well, some not too well. Trials will come and go if we handle them properly. At the end of every trial there should be some growth. It is true that we can't be happy all the time, but making a commitment to pursue happiness can do some good to prepare us for the bad days ahead. Happiness is a state of mind that exists when you are surrounded by people who love you and you love in return. Many experience that love from their grandchildren. I once saw a bumper sticker that said: If I knew that grandchildren would be so much fun, I would have had them first. These people are expressing wellness and joy, rather than loneliness and depression.

Over the years, I have received many gifts. The ones that I treasure the most are the ones from family especially my grand-children. For Mother's Day 2018, I got a card from my grand-children which said on the front cover: "Grandma" is just another word for "love". On the inside it said,

You know, like 'grandchild' is just another word for "cutest kid on the face of the earth". This surely raised my vibration to a ten. I keep cards like this one in plain view where I can see it. Quite often, I re-read all these precious gifts to express my wellness and joy. As you can see, the best things in life are free. Enjoy every minute and cherish every good memory. You will in return have sunshine in the midst of the dark clouds.

Friendships are cultivated from people we've met and known over the years. From the time we start school, we start meeting people. Just think, if we keep and maintain one friend from every school grade and every work place, the number of friends we would have. Memories and imaginations never wear out. Cherish the ones that make you chuckle and smile when you think of them. I have come to realise that every person in my life is there for a reason. Those that have dropped off are no longer needed, for they have accomplished what needed to be done in me.

What will we be remembered for?

I want to be remembered for my faith in God. As I get older, I find that my faith grows along with me. Not old, but strong. I have the confidence to do more than when I was younger. I did not become an artist, but I have many artistic abilities. I have the boldness to share tips and ideas that may be helpful to others, especially the young. That comes from notes gathered over the years. I have the courage to say No to tasks demanded of me that put too much pressure on me. Saying 'No' was forced upon me. Now I cherish the process that pushed me to learn from it.

Mary Abdool-Warner

I try to spend time with people who inspire or uplift me. I wish I knew that when I was younger.

I would have written this book years before now. I no longer try to help those who do not want my help. I focus on those who need my help.

The most liberating thing that I learned is to be myself. It does not matter what others think or say about me. I know whose I am. I am a child of God. I am fearfully and wonderfully made. Psalm 139: 14. It is no secret what God can do with a life that surrenders to Him. I constantly remind myself of a song I learned many years ago which says:

> I am a Promise,
> I am a Possibility,
> I am a Promise
> With a capital "P"
> I am a great big bundle of POTENTIALITY
> And if I listen, I'll hear God's voice
> And if I'm trying
> He'll help me make the right choice
> For I'm a Promise to be
> Everything God wants me to be.

One of the things we learn as we get older is, we need less. We need much less than we think we need. How many pairs of shoes do we need? How many purses and bags do we need? How many outfits do we need? We need far less than we own. Do we need to have the latest gadget on the market? In most cases we don't. Over the years, I've watched my daughters purge out their closets at least twice a year. Did they really need those things when they purchased them?

Those who have experienced 'Near Death Experience' all return with a new mandate to live life to the fullest. They aim to create heaven on earth by viewing all people as having worth and full of potential. They feel a greater sense of purpose for their lives. Former criminals are transformed to counsellors to help troubled youths. Workaholics become loving and caring to their families. The impatient and short-tempered become easy going and tolerant. Even the materialistic become wise spenders. During their experiences, they experienced feeling of no judgment, only overwhelming unconditional love. As Anita Moorjani in her book "Dying to be Me" says, there was a sense of universal understanding and knowledge. Now they practice gratitude for ALL that transpires in their lives. They make choices fuelled by passion and love.

They conclude that nothing happens by accident and there is no such thing as coincidence.

During our time here, we all have something to overcome. In many cases it is a challenge to help us grow. Worry, low self-esteem, anger, pride, greed, addiction, fear and negative thinking are some of the personal problems that can control us and keep us from true happiness. These things are written by those who experienced Near Death, to teach us how to live before we die, never to return in our present state of being.

Bibliography

Dr. Axe, Josh. "Keto Diet: Your 30-Day Plan to Lose Weight, Balance Hormones, Boost Brain."

https://draxe.com.

Batt, Sharon. "Be Aware of Who is Funding Breast Cancer Campaigns." The Toronto Star, October 11,2017.

Bollinger, Charlene and Ty. "The Truth About Cancer." https://thetruthaboutcancer.com.

Dr. Dispenza, Joe. "You Are the Placebo: Making Your Mind Matter." New York: Hay House Inc. April 2014.

Eden, Donna. "Donna Eden's Daily Energy Routine." DonnaEden.com, You Tube November 24, 2015.

Dr. Emoto, Masaru. "Water, Consciousness and Intent." Purpleleisureologist, Published March 13, 2009.

Dr. Fung, Jason. "The Perfect treatment for Diabetes and Weight Loss." https://www.dietdoctor.com/the perf. You Tube May 9, 2015.

Dr. Gerson, Max. "Nutritional Cancer Therapy." (Max, B. 1881-1959) https://www.emedicinehealth.com/gerson_therapy/article_em.htm.

Hay, Louise L. "You Can Heal Your Life." You Tube November 14, 2018. https://www.Amazon.ca/You-Can-Heal-Your-Life.

Moorjani, Anita. "Dying to be Me." New York: Hay House Inc. 2012.

Philip, Darryl J. "Relax: You're Not going to Die. Part 1." Canada: First Spirit Publishing Inc. 2016.

Dr. Quiillin, Patrick. "Beating Cancer with Nutrition." http://getting healthier.com.

Dr. Seyfreid, Thomas. "Cancer as a Metabolic Disease." Wiley Press, February 19, 2015.

Hays, Tom and Long, Colleen. "Pharma Bro' Shkreli gets seven years in Prison." The Toronto Star, March 10, 2018.

Wark, Chris. "How I Used the Raw Vegan Diet to Beat Cancer." https://chrisbeat cancer.com/the-raw-vegan-diet/.

Wayne, Debora. "Why Do I Still Hurt?: Rapid Relief of Chronic Pain." https://www.amazon.com/Why-Do-Still-Hurt-Depression-ebook/dp/BO196 5QGOS.

Winters, Nasha. "The Metabolic Approach to Cancer: Integrating Deep Nutrition, The Ketogenic Diet, and Non-toxic Bio-Individualized Therapies." You Tube May 24, 2017.

Dr. Zielinski, Eric. "Beat Cancer God's Way: Learn God's Victorious Blueprint." https://naturallivingfamily.com/How-to-beat-cancer-god's-way.

About the Author

Mary was born in a little village called Micoud, one of the villages that make up the island of Saint Lucia. It reminds her of the little village of Nazareth from the bible, where a disciple, before he became a disciple of Jesus Christ said, "Can anything good come from Nazareth?" (John 1:46) Well, because of the size, some may be asking the same question about Micoud. Yes, something good came out of Micoud. Mary visited Israel in February 2012, and found it to be hilly, mountainous and lush with palm trees just the way it is described in the bible.

For as long as Mary can remember, she'd always wanted to be a teacher. Yes, remember what your child says from a young age what he or she wants to be. Our job as parents is to gently guide them in that direction. It may well be that that is their gift or calling in life. At a very young age, Mary wanted to be a teacher. She modelled her teachers and played school, pretending to teach a class of children. They did not have paper and pen to write with in those days. They had what was called a slate to write on and chalk to write with. It did its job then. She ended up teaching right after finishing high school for real, not pretend. She left that teaching position to migrate to Canada, where she met and married her children's father. They have two daughters, seven grandchildren and three great-grandchildren.

Printed in the United States
By Bookmasters